TYPE 1 DIABETES VEGETARIAN MEAL PLAN FOR WEIGHT LOSS

Delicious Recipes for Balanced Blood Sugar & Sustainable Weight Management

By Mia Bennett

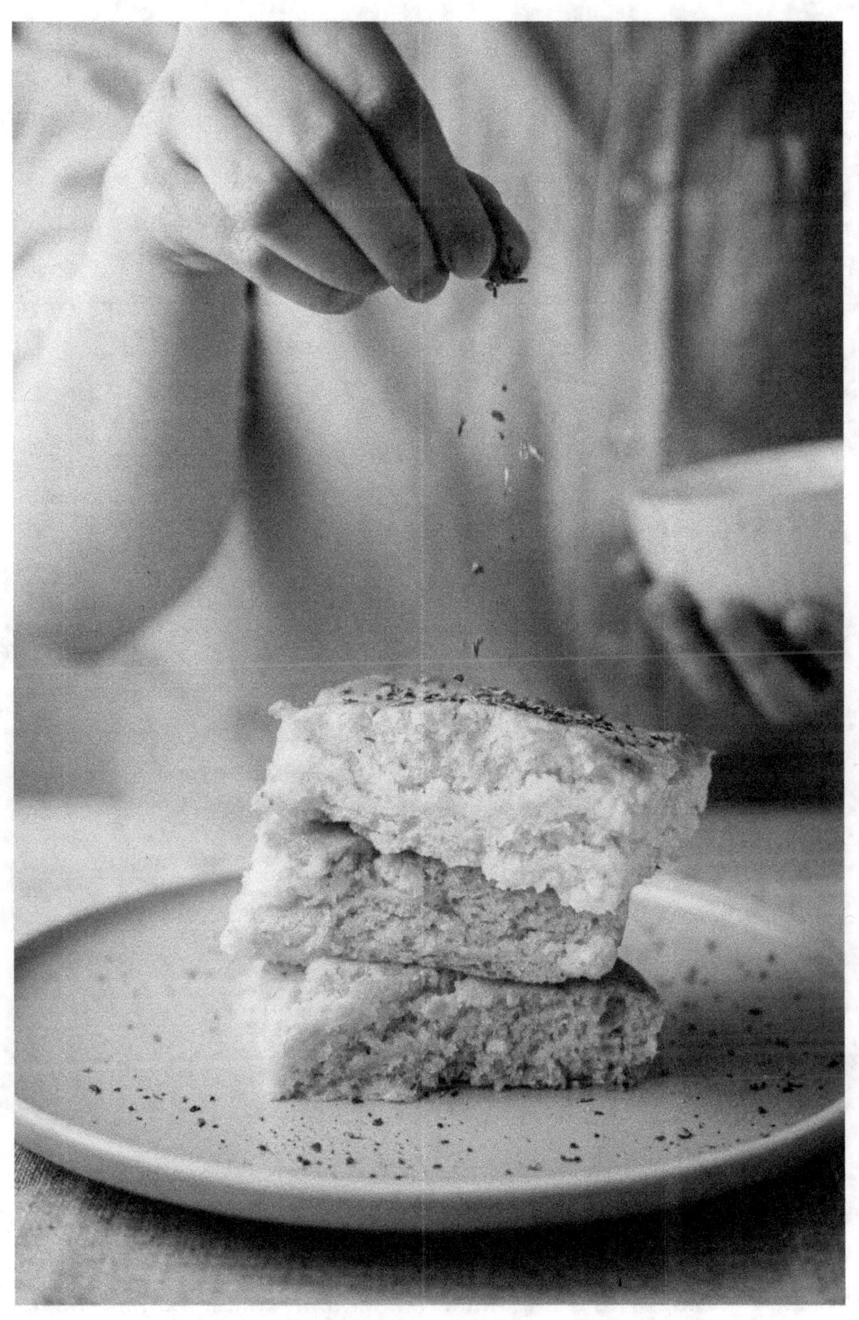

TABLE OF CONTENTS

Chapter 3: Lunch Recipes 39

Chapter 4: Dinner Recipes 58

CONCLUSION 124

INTRODUCTION

Living with diabetes can feel overwhelming at times, but knowledge is a powerful tool. This guide dives into understanding Type 1 diabetes, the crucial role of diet in managing it, and explores how a vegetarian approach can contribute to weight loss goals.

Understanding Type 1 Diabetes:

Unlike Type 2 diabetes, where the body struggles to use insulin effectively, Type 1 is an autoimmune condition. The body's immune system mistakenly attacks the insulin-producing cells in the pancreas, leaving you unable to produce insulin. Insulin acts like a key, unlocking the door for glucose (sugar) from your bloodstream to enter your cells and be used for energy. Without enough insulin, glucose builds up in the bloodstream, leading to a variety of health concerns.

The Dietary Dance:

Diet becomes an essential partner in managing Type 1 diabetes. Food choices directly impact blood sugar levels. Carbohydrates, in particular, are broken down into glucose, so understanding how different foods affect your blood sugar is key. Here's where things get interesting: a registered dietitian can help you create a personalized plan that factors in your activity level, insulin dosage, and preferences. It's not about deprivation, but about embracing a balanced approach that includes:

- **Colorful Veggies**: They're packed with essential nutrients and have minimal impact on blood sugar. Think leafy greens, broccoli, peppers, and whatever tickles your taste buds.
- **Fiber-Rich Choices:** Whole grains, legumes, and nuts provide sustained energy and help regulate blood sugar levels.
- **Lean Protein Sources**: Fish, chicken, tofu, and beans keep you feeling full and provide essential building blocks for your body.
- **Healthy Fats:** Avocados, nuts, and olive oil promote satiety and offer essential nutrients.

Vegetarian Options and Weight Management:

A well-planned vegetarian diet can be incredibly beneficial for managing Type 1 diabetes and weight loss. Here's why:

- **Fiber Powerhouse:** Vegetarian meals are often naturally high in fiber, promoting gut health and keeping you feeling fuller for longer, reducing calorie intake.

- **Weight Management Ally:** Studies suggest vegetarian diets can be helpful for weight loss, which can significantly improve blood sugar control in Type 1 diabetes.

- **Nutrient Rich:** A well-planned vegetarian diet can be brimming with essential vitamins, minerals, and antioxidants, promoting overall health.

Goals for Weight Loss:

Weight loss can be a significant factor in managing Type 1 diabetes. Even modest weight loss can improve insulin sensitivity and make blood sugar control easier. Here are some realistic and sustainable weight loss goals:

- **Small, Steady Steps:** Aim for a weight loss of 1-2 pounds per week. Slow and steady wins the race, especially when it comes to long-term lifestyle changes.

- **Focus on Habits:** Instead of crash diets, focus on building healthy habits like portion control, mindful eating, and incorporating regular physical activity.

Remember, you're not alone on this journey. With a good understanding of Type 1 diabetes, the power of diet in managing it, and the potential benefits of a vegetarian approach, you can create a healthy lifestyle that supports your weight loss goals and overall well-being.

Chapter 1: 30 Day Meal Plan

Week 1

Day 1

- Breakfast: Avocado Toast with Cherry Tomatoes
- Lunch: Lentil and Veggie Soup
- Dinner: Eggplant Parmesan
- Snack: Roasted Chickpeas
- Dessert: Baked Apples with Cinnamon

Day 2

- Breakfast: Veggie-Packed Scrambled Tofu
- Lunch: Chickpea Salad with Tahini Dressing
- Dinner: Chickpea and Spinach Stew
- Snack: Veggie Sticks with Hummus
- Dessert: Chia Seed Pudding with Coconut Milk

Day 3

- Breakfast: Greek Yogurt with Berries and Chia Seeds
- Lunch: Grilled Veggie Wrap
- Dinner: Stuffed Acorn Squash
- Snack: Edamame with Sea Salt
- Dessert: Dark Chocolate Avocado Mousse

Day 4

- Breakfast: Overnight Oats with Almond Milk and Fresh Fruit
- Lunch: Spinach and Quinoa Salad with Lemon Vinaigrette
- Dinner: Tofu Stir-Fry with Brown Rice
- Snack: Baked Zucchini Fries
- Dessert: Berry Sorbet

Day 5

- Breakfast: Spinach and Mushroom Omelette
- Lunch: Tomato Basil Soup with Whole Grain Croutons
- Dinner: Spaghetti Squash with Marinara Sauce
- Snack: Spicy Roasted Almonds
- Dessert: Almond Flour Brownies

Day 6

- Breakfast: Quinoa Breakfast Bowl with Nuts and Seeds
- Lunch: Roasted Vegetable Buddha Bowl
- Dinner: Vegetable Paella
- Snack: Cucumber Rolls with Avocado and Tomato
- Dessert: Coconut Macaroons

Day 7

- Breakfast: Apple Cinnamon Porridge

- Lunch: Black Bean and Corn Salad
- Dinner: Baked Ziti with Ricotta and Spinach
- Snack: Greek Yogurt Dip with Veggies
- Dessert: Date and Nut Energy Balls

Week 2

Day 8

- Breakfast: Protein-Packed Smoothie Bowl
- Lunch: Mediterranean Stuffed Peppers
- Dinner: Thai Peanut Tofu Bowl
- Snack: Mini Caprese Skewers
- Dessert: Vegan Cheesecake with Cashew Cream

Day 9

- Breakfast: Baked Sweet Potato and Black Bean Breakfast Burrito
- Lunch: Zucchini Noodles with Pesto
- Dinner: Veggie-Loaded Burrito Bowl
- Snack: Stuffed Mini Bell Peppers
- Dessert: Apple Crisp with Oats

Day 10

- Breakfast: Whole Wheat Pancakes with Berry Compote

- Lunch: Spicy Tofu Lettuce Wraps
- Dinner: Lentil Shepherd's Pie
- Snack: Guacamole with Celery Sticks
- Dessert: Mango Sticky Rice

Day 11

- Breakfast: Chia Pudding with Mango
- Lunch: Cauliflower Rice Sushi Rolls
- Dinner: Mushroom Stroganoff
- Snack: Kale Chips
- Dessert: Peanut Butter Banana Ice Cream

Day 12

- Breakfast: Savory Breakfast Muffins with Veggies
- Lunch: Kale and White Bean Stew
- Dinner: Cauliflower Tacos with Cilantro Lime Sauce
- Snack: Apple Slices with Almond Butter
- Dessert: Oatmeal Raisin Cookies

Day 13

- Breakfast: Cottage Cheese and Peach Bowl
- Lunch: Cucumber and Avocado Salad
- Dinner: Spinach and Feta Stuffed Portobellos
- Snack: Tofu Bites with Sweet Chili Sauce

- Dessert: Fruit Salad with Lime and Mint

Day 14

- Breakfast: Buckwheat Groats with Almond Butter and Banana
- Lunch: Mushroom and Barley Risotto
- Dinner: Butternut Squash and Chickpea Tagine
- Snack: Carrot and Raisin Salad
- Dessert: Chocolate Covered Strawberries

Week 3

Day 15

- Breakfast: Green Smoothie with Spinach, Banana, and Protein Powder
- Lunch: Sweet Potato and Lentil Curry
- Dinner: Grilled Vegetable and Quinoa Skewers
- Snack: Stuffed Grape Leaves
- Dessert: Lemon Poppy Seed Muffins

Day 16

- Breakfast: Avocado Toast with Cherry Tomatoes
- Lunch: Lentil and Veggie Soup
- Dinner: Eggplant Parmesan

- Snack: Roasted Chickpeas
- Dessert: Baked Apples with Cinnamon

Day 17

- Breakfast: Veggie-Packed Scrambled Tofu
- Lunch: Chickpea Salad with Tahini Dressing
- Dinner: Chickpea and Spinach Stew
- Snack: Veggie Sticks with Hummus
- Dessert: Chia Seed Pudding with Coconut Milk

Day 18

- Breakfast: Greek Yogurt with Berries and Chia Seeds
- Lunch: Grilled Veggie Wrap
- Dinner: Stuffed Acorn Squash
- Snack: Edamame with Sea Salt
- Dessert: Dark Chocolate Avocado Mousse

Day 19

- Breakfast: Overnight Oats with Almond Milk and Fresh Fruit
- Lunch: Spinach and Quinoa Salad with Lemon Vinaigrette
- Dinner: Tofu Stir-Fry with Brown Rice
- Snack: Baked Zucchini Fries
- Dessert: Berry Sorbet

Day 20

- Breakfast: Spinach and Mushroom Omelette
- Lunch: Tomato Basil Soup with Whole Grain Croutons
- Dinner: Spaghetti Squash with Marinara Sauce
- Snack: Spicy Roasted Almonds
- Dessert: Almond Flour Brownies

Day 21

- Breakfast: Quinoa Breakfast Bowl with Nuts and Seeds
- Lunch: Roasted Vegetable Buddha Bowl
- Dinner: Vegetable Paella
- Snack: Cucumber Rolls with Avocado and Tomato
- Dessert: Coconut Macaroons

Week 4

Day 22

- Breakfast: Apple Cinnamon Porridge
- Lunch: Black Bean and Corn Salad
- Dinner: Baked Ziti with Ricotta and Spinach
- Snack: Greek Yogurt Dip with Veggies
- Dessert: Date and Nut Energy Balls

Day 23

- Breakfast: Protein-Packed Smoothie Bowl
- Lunch: Mediterranean Stuffed Peppers
- Dinner: Thai Peanut Tofu Bowl
- Snack: Mini Caprese Skewers
- Dessert: Vegan Cheesecake with Cashew Cream

Day 24

- Breakfast: Baked Sweet Potato and Black Bean Breakfast Burrito
- Lunch: Zucchini Noodles with Pesto
- Dinner: Veggie-Loaded Burrito Bowl
- Snack: Stuffed Mini Bell Peppers
- Dessert: Apple Crisp with Oats

Day 25

- Breakfast: Whole Wheat Pancakes with Berry Compote
- Lunch: Spicy Tofu Lettuce Wraps
- Dinner: Lentil Shepherd's Pie
- Snack: Guacamole with Celery Sticks
- Dessert: Mango Sticky Rice

Day 26

- Breakfast: Chia Pudding with Mango

- Lunch: Cauliflower Rice Sushi Rolls
- Dinner: Mushroom Stroganoff
- Snack: Kale Chips
- Dessert: Peanut Butter Banana Ice Cream

Day 27

- Breakfast: Savory Breakfast Muffins with Veggies
- Lunch: Kale and White Bean Stew
- Dinner: Cauliflower Tacos with Cilantro Lime Sauce
- Snack: Apple Slices with Almond Butter
- Dessert: Oatmeal Raisin Cookies

Day 28

- Breakfast: Cottage Cheese and Peach Bowl
- Lunch: Cucumber and Avocado Salad
- Dinner: Spinach and Feta Stuffed Portobellos
- Snack: Tofu Bites with Sweet Chili Sauce
- Dessert: Fruit Salad with Lime and Mint

Day 29

- Breakfast: Buckwheat Groats with Almond Butter and Banana
- Lunch: Mushroom and Barley Risotto
- Dinner: Butternut Squash and Chickpea Tagine

- Snack: Carrot and Raisin Salad

- Dessert: Chocolate Covered Strawberries

Day 30

- Breakfast: Green Smoothie with Spinach, Banana, and Protein Powder

- Lunch: Sweet Potato and Lentil Curry

- Dinner: Grilled Vegetable and Quinoa Skewers

- Snack: Stuffed Grape Leaves

- Dessert: Lemon Poppy Seed Muffins

Chapter 2: Breakfast Recipes

Starting your day with a nutritious and balanced breakfast is essential, especially for individuals managing Type 1 diabetes. These vegetarian recipes are designed to be both satisfying and supportive of weight loss goals, offering a variety of flavors and nutrients to keep you energized throughout the morning.

Avocado Toast with Cherry Tomatoes

Ingredients:

- 1 slice of whole grain bread, toasted
- 1/2 avocado, mashed
- 5 cherry tomatoes, halved
- Salt and pepper to taste
- 1 tsp olive oil (optional)

Instructions:

1. Spread the mashed avocado evenly on the toasted bread.
2. Top with cherry tomatoes.
3. Season with salt and pepper. Drizzle with olive oil if desired.

Nutrition Information:

- Calories: 200

- Protein: 4g

- Carbohydrates: 20g

- Fat: 14g

- Fiber: 8g

- Sugar: 2g

- Portion Size: 1 slice

Veggie-Packed Scrambled Tofu

Ingredients:

- 1/2 block firm tofu, crumbled

- 1/4 cup bell peppers, diced

- 1/4 cup spinach, chopped

- 1/4 cup onion, diced

- 1 tbsp olive oil

- 1/2 tsp turmeric

- Salt and pepper to taste

Instructions:

1. Heat olive oil in a pan over medium heat.

2. Add onions and bell peppers, sauté until softened.

3. Add crumbled tofu and turmeric, cook for 5 minutes.

4. Stir in spinach, cook until wilted.

5. Season with salt and pepper.

Nutrition Information:

- Calories: 180
- Protein: 12g
- Carbohydrates: 8g
- Fat: 12g
- Fiber: 3g
- Sugar: 2g
- Portion Size: 1 serving

Greek Yogurt with Berries and Chia Seeds

Ingredients:

- 1 cup Greek yogurt
- 1/2 cup mixed berries
- 1 tbsp chia seeds
- 1 tsp honey (optional)

Instructions:

1. In a bowl, combine Greek yogurt and mixed berries.
2. Sprinkle chia seeds on top.
3. Drizzle with honey if desired.

Nutrition Information:

- Calories: 200
- Protein: 15g
- Carbohydrates: 20g
- Fat: 5g
- Fiber: 5g
- Sugar: 15g
- Portion Size: 1 bowl

Overnight Oats with Almond Milk and Fresh Fruit

Ingredients:

- 1/2 cup rolled oats
- 1/2 cup almond milk
- 1/4 cup fresh fruit (e.g., berries, banana slices)
- 1 tbsp chia seeds

Instructions:

1. In a jar, combine oats, almond milk, and chia seeds.
2. Stir well and refrigerate overnight.
3. Top with fresh fruit before serving.

Nutrition Information:

- Calories: 250
- Protein: 8g
- Carbohydrates: 40g
- Fat: 7g
- Fiber: 8g
- Sugar: 10g
- Portion Size: 1 jar

Spinach and Mushroom Omelette

Ingredients:

- 2 eggs
- 1/4 cup spinach, chopped
- 1/4 cup mushrooms, sliced
- 1 tbsp olive oil
- Salt and pepper to taste

Instructions:

1. Heat olive oil in a pan over medium heat.
2. Sauté mushrooms until soft, then add spinach and cook until wilted.
3. Beat eggs and pour into the pan, cooking until set.
4. Fold omelette and season with salt and pepper.

Nutrition Information:

- Calories: 210
- Protein: 14g
- Carbohydrates: 4g
- Fat: 16g
- Fiber: 2g
- Sugar: 1g
- Portion Size: 1 omelette

Quinoa Breakfast Bowl with Nuts and Seeds

Ingredients:

- 1/2 cup cooked quinoa
- 1/4 cup mixed nuts (e.g., almonds, walnuts)
- 1 tbsp pumpkin seeds
- 1 tbsp honey
- 1/4 cup almond milk

Instructions:

1. Combine cooked quinoa, mixed nuts, and pumpkin seeds in a bowl.
2. Drizzle with honey and pour over almond milk.

Nutrition Information:

- Calories: 350
- Protein: 10g
- Carbohydrates: 40g
- Fat: 18g
- Fiber: 7g
- Sugar: 10g
- Portion Size: 1 bowl

Apple Cinnamon Porridge

Ingredients:

- 1/2 cup rolled oats
- 1 cup water
- 1/2 apple, diced
- 1/2 tsp cinnamon
- 1 tsp maple syrup (optional)

Instructions:

1. In a pot, combine oats, water, apple, and cinnamon.
2. Cook over medium heat until oats are soft.
3. Drizzle with maple syrup if desired.

Nutrition Information:

- Calories: 180
- Protein: 5g
- Carbohydrates: 34g
- Fat: 3g
- Fiber: 5g
- Sugar: 10g
- Portion Size: 1 bowl

Protein-Packed Smoothie Bowl

Ingredients:

- 1 banana
- 1/2 cup Greek yogurt
- 1/2 cup spinach
- 1 tbsp almond butter
- 1 tbsp chia seeds
- 1/2 cup almond milk

Instructions:

1. Blend all ingredients until smooth.
2. Pour into a bowl and top with additional chia seeds or fruit if desired.

Nutrition Information:

- Calories: 300
- Protein: 15g
- Carbohydrates: 35g
- Fat: 12g
- Fiber: 8g
- Sugar: 15g
- Portion Size: 1 bowl

Baked Sweet Potato and Black Bean Breakfast Burrito

Ingredients:

- 1 small sweet potato, diced
- 1/2 cup black beans
- 1 whole grain tortilla
- 1/4 avocado, sliced
- 1 tbsp salsa

Instructions:

1. Bake sweet potato at 400°F for 20 minutes or until soft.
2. In a tortilla, combine sweet potato, black beans, avocado, and salsa.
3. Roll up and serve warm.

Nutrition Information:

- Calories: 350
- Protein: 12g
- Carbohydrates: 55g
- Fat: 10g
- Fiber: 14g
- Sugar: 7g
- Portion Size: 1 burrito

Whole Wheat Pancakes with Berry Compote

Ingredients:

- 1 cup whole wheat flour
- 1 cup almond milk
- 1 egg
- 1 tsp baking powder
- 1 cup mixed berries
- 1 tbsp honey

Instructions:

1. Mix flour, almond milk, egg, and baking powder until smooth.
2. Cook pancakes on a griddle until bubbles form, then flip.

3. For the compote, heat berries and honey in a saucepan until soft.

4. Serve pancakes topped with berry compote.

Nutrition Information:

- Calories: 300
- Protein: 10g
- Carbohydrates: 50g
- Fat: 6g
- Fiber: 8g
- Sugar: 15g
- Portion Size: 2 pancakes

Chia Pudding with Mango

Ingredients:

- 1/4 cup chia seeds
- 1 cup almond milk
- 1/2 mango, diced
- 1 tsp maple syrup (optional)

Instructions:

1. Combine chia seeds and almond milk in a jar.

2. Stir well and refrigerate overnight.

3. Top with diced mango and maple syrup if desired.

Nutrition Information:

- Calories: 250
- Protein: 6g
- Carbohydrates: 32g
- Fat: 12g
- Fiber: 10g
- Sugar: 18g
- Portion Size: 1 jar

Savory Breakfast Muffins with Veggies

Ingredients:

- 1 cup whole wheat flour
- 1/2 cup milk
- 2 eggs
- 1/2 cup spinach, chopped
- 1/4 cup bell peppers, diced
- 1/4 cup cheese, shredded (optional)
- 1 tsp baking powder
- Salt and pepper to taste

Instructions:

1. Preheat oven to 375°F.

2. Mix all ingredients in a bowl.

3. Spoon batter into muffin tin and bake for 20 minutes.

Nutrition Information:

- Calories: 150

- Protein: 7g

- Carbohydrates: 18g

- Fat: 6g

- Fiber: 3g

- Sugar: 2g

- Portion Size: 1 muffin

Cottage Cheese and Peach Bowl

Ingredients:

- 1 cup cottage cheese

- 1 peach, sliced

- 1 tbsp honey

- 1 tbsp flax seeds

Instructions:

1. In a bowl, combine cottage cheese and peach slices.

2. Drizzle with honey and sprinkle with flax seeds.

Nutrition Information:

- Calories: 220
- Protein: 15g
- Carbohydrates: 25g
- Fat: 7g
- Fiber: 4g
- Sugar: 18g
- Portion Size: 1 bowl

Buckwheat Groats with Almond Butter and Banana

Ingredients:

- 1/2 cup buckwheat groats
- 1 cup water
- 1 banana, sliced
- 1 tbsp almond butter

Instructions:

1. Cook buckwheat groats in water over medium heat until tender.
2. Top with sliced banana and almond butter.

Nutrition Information:

- Calories: 300
- Protein: 8g
- Carbohydrates: 50g
- Fat: 10g
- Fiber: 8g
- Sugar: 12g
- Portion Size: 1 bowl

Green Smoothie with Spinach, Banana, and Protein Powder

Ingredients:

- 1 banana
- 1 cup spinach
- 1 scoop protein powder
- 1 cup almond milk
- 1 tbsp chia seeds

Instructions:

1. Blend all ingredients until smooth.
2. Pour into a glass and serve immediately.

Nutrition Information:

- Calories: 250
- Protein: 20g
- Carbohydrates: 30g
- Fat: 8g
- Fiber: 6g
- Sugar: 15g
- Portion Size: 1 glass

Chapter 3: Lunch Recipes

A well-balanced lunch is essential for maintaining energy levels and managing blood sugar, especially for individuals with Type 1 diabetes. These vegetarian lunch recipes are designed to be nutritious, delicious, and conducive to weight loss.

Lentil and Veggie Soup

Ingredients:

- 1 cup lentils, rinsed
- 1 onion, diced
- 2 carrots, chopped
- 2 celery stalks, chopped
- 3 garlic cloves, minced
- 1 zucchini, chopped
- 1 can diced tomatoes
- 6 cups vegetable broth
- 1 tsp cumin
- 1 tsp thyme
- Salt and pepper to taste
- 2 tbsp olive oil

Instructions:

1. In a large pot, heat olive oil over medium heat.
2. Add onion, carrots, celery, and garlic, sauté until soft.
3. Add lentils, zucchini, diced tomatoes, and vegetable broth.
4. Season with cumin, thyme, salt, and pepper.
5. Bring to a boil, then reduce heat and simmer for 30 minutes, or until lentils are tender.

Nutrition Information (per serving):

- Calories: 250
- Protein: 12g
- Carbohydrates: 40g
- Fat: 6g
- Fiber: 15g
- Sugar: 7g
- Portion Size: 1 bowl (about 2 cups)

Chickpea Salad with Tahini Dressing

Ingredients:

- 1 can chickpeas, rinsed and drained
- 1 cucumber, diced
- 1 bell pepper, diced
- 1/2 red onion, finely chopped

- 1/4 cup chopped parsley
- 2 tbsp tahini
- 1 lemon, juiced
- 1 tbsp olive oil
- Salt and pepper to taste

Instructions:

1. In a large bowl, combine chickpeas, cucumber, bell pepper, red onion, and parsley.
2. In a small bowl, whisk together tahini, lemon juice, olive oil, salt, and pepper.
3. Pour the dressing over the salad and toss to combine.

Nutrition Information (per serving):

- Calories: 220
- Protein: 8g
- Carbohydrates: 25g
- Fat: 10g
- Fiber: 8g
- Sugar: 5g
- Portion Size: 1 cup

Grilled Veggie Wrap

Ingredients:

- 1 whole wheat tortilla
- 1/2 zucchini, sliced
- 1/2 eggplant, sliced
- 1/2 bell pepper, sliced
- 1/4 cup hummus
- Handful of spinach leaves
- 1 tbsp olive oil
- Salt and pepper to taste

Instructions:

1. Brush zucchini, eggplant, and bell pepper with olive oil, season with salt and pepper.
2. Grill the vegetables on medium heat until tender and slightly charred.
3. Spread hummus on the tortilla, layer with grilled vegetables and spinach.
4. Roll up the tortilla, slice in half, and serve.

Nutrition Information (per serving):

- Calories: 280
- Protein: 8g
- Carbohydrates: 35g

- Fat: 12g

- Fiber: 8g

- Sugar: 5g

- Portion Size: 1 wrap

Spinach and Quinoa Salad with Lemon Vinaigrette

Ingredients:

- 1 cup cooked quinoa

- 2 cups fresh spinach leaves

- 1/2 cup cherry tomatoes, halved

- 1/4 red onion, thinly sliced

- 1/4 cup feta cheese, crumbled

- 1/4 cup walnuts, chopped

- Juice of 1 lemon

- 2 tbsp olive oil

- Salt and pepper to taste

Instructions:

1. In a large bowl, combine quinoa, spinach, cherry tomatoes, red onion, feta, and walnuts.

2. In a small bowl, whisk together lemon juice, olive oil, salt, and pepper.

3. Pour the dressing over the salad and toss to combine.

Nutrition Information (per serving):

- Calories: 300
- Protein: 10g
- Carbohydrates: 25g
- Fat: 18g
- Fiber: 5g
- Sugar: 3g
- Portion Size: 1.5 cups

Tomato Basil Soup with Whole Grain Croutons

Ingredients:

- 6 ripe tomatoes, chopped
- 1 onion, chopped
- 3 garlic cloves, minced
- 2 cups vegetable broth
- 1/4 cup fresh basil leaves, chopped
- 2 tbsp olive oil
- Salt and pepper to taste
- 2 slices whole grain bread, cubed

Instructions:

1. In a large pot, heat olive oil over medium heat. Sauté onion and garlic until soft.
2. Add tomatoes and vegetable broth, bring to a boil. Reduce heat and simmer for 20 minutes.
3. Blend the soup until smooth, season with salt, pepper, and stir in basil.
4. For croutons, toast bread cubes in a dry skillet until crispy.
5. Serve the soup topped with croutons.

Nutrition Information (per serving):

- Calories: 220
- Protein: 5g
- Carbohydrates: 30g
- Fat: 10g
- Fiber: 6g
- Sugar: 10g
- Portion Size: 1 bowl (about 1.5 cups)

Roasted Vegetable Buddha Bowl

Ingredients:

- 1 cup cooked brown rice
- 1/2 cup roasted sweet potato cubes

- 1/2 cup roasted broccoli florets
- 1/2 cup roasted chickpeas
- 1/4 avocado, sliced
- 2 tbsp tahini
- 1 lemon, juiced
- Salt and pepper to taste

Instructions:

1. Assemble brown rice, roasted sweet potato, broccoli, and chickpeas in a bowl.
2. Top with avocado slices.
3. In a small bowl, whisk together tahini, lemon juice, salt, and pepper.
4. Drizzle dressing over the bowl and serve.

Nutrition Information (per serving):

- Calories: 350
- Protein: 10g
- Carbohydrates: 45g
- Fat: 15g
- Fiber: 10g
- Sugar: 5g
- Portion Size: 1 bowl

Black Bean and Corn Salad

Ingredients:

- 1 can black beans, rinsed and drained
- 1 cup corn kernels
- 1 red bell pepper, diced
- 1/4 red onion, finely chopped
- 1/4 cup cilantro, chopped
- Juice of 1 lime
- 2 tbsp olive oil
- Salt and pepper to taste

Instructions:

1. In a large bowl, combine black beans, corn, bell pepper, red onion, and cilantro.
2. In a small bowl, whisk together lime juice, olive oil, salt, and pepper.
3. Pour dressing over the salad and toss to combine.

Nutrition Information (per serving):

- Calories: 220
- Protein: 8g
- Carbohydrates: 32g
- Fat: 8g
- Fiber: 10g

- Sugar: 5g
- Portion Size: 1 cup

Mediterranean Stuffed Peppers

Ingredients:

- 4 bell peppers, halved and seeded
- 1 cup cooked quinoa
- 1/2 cup chickpeas
- 1/4 cup kalamata olives, sliced
- 1/4 cup feta cheese, crumbled
- 1/4 cup parsley, chopped
- 2 tbsp olive oil
- 1 tsp oregano
- Salt and pepper to taste

Instructions:

1. Preheat oven to 375°F (190°C).
2. In a bowl, combine quinoa, chickpeas, olives, feta, parsley, olive oil, oregano, salt, and pepper.
3. Stuff bell pepper halves with the mixture.
4. Place peppers in a baking dish and bake for 30 minutes.

Nutrition Information (per serving):

- Calories: 250
- Protein: 9g
- Carbohydrates: 28g
- Fat: 12g
- Fiber: 7g
- Sugar: 6g
- Portion Size: 2 stuffed pepper halves

Zucchini Noodles with Pesto

Ingredients:

- 2 large zucchinis, spiralized
- 1 cup cherry tomatoes, halved
- 1/4 cup pesto
- 2 tbsp pine nuts, toasted
- 1 tbsp olive oil
- Salt and pepper to taste

Instructions:

1. Heat olive oil in a large pan over medium heat.
2. Add zucchini noodles and cook for 2-3 minutes until slightly softened.

3. Remove from heat, toss with pesto, cherry tomatoes, pine nuts, salt, and pepper.

4. Serve immediately.

Nutrition Information (per serving):

- Calories: 200

- Protein: 5g

- Carbohydrates: 10g

- Fat: 16g

- Fiber: 3g

- Sugar: 5g

- Portion Size: 1.5 cups

Spicy Tofu Lettuce Wraps

Ingredients:

- 1 block firm tofu, crumbled

- 1 carrot, grated

- 1/2 bell pepper, diced

- 2 green onions, chopped

- 2 tbsp soy sauce

- 1 tbsp sriracha

- 1 tbsp sesame oil

- Lettuce leaves

Instructions:

1. In a pan, heat sesame oil over medium heat. Add tofu, carrot, and bell pepper.
2. Stir in soy sauce and sriracha, cook for 5-7 minutes.
3. Spoon mixture into lettuce leaves, top with green onions, and serve.

Nutrition Information (per serving):

- Calories: 220
- Protein: 12g
- Carbohydrates: 10g
- Fat: 15g
- Fiber: 4g
- Sugar: 5g
- Portion Size: 3 wraps

Cauliflower Rice Sushi Rolls

Ingredients:

- 1 head cauliflower, riced
- 1 avocado, sliced
- 1 cucumber, julienned
- 1 carrot, julienned
- 1 sheet nori

- 2 tbsp rice vinegar
- Soy sauce for serving

Instructions:

1. In a pan, cook riced cauliflower over medium heat for 5 minutes. Stir in rice vinegar.
2. Lay nori on a sushi mat, spread cauliflower rice evenly.
3. Layer with avocado, cucumber, and carrot.
4. Roll tightly and slice into pieces. Serve with soy sauce.

Nutrition Information (per serving):

- Calories: 180
- Protein: 4g
- Carbohydrates: 15g
- Fat: 12g
- Fiber: 7g
- Sugar: 4g
- Portion Size: 1 roll

Kale and White Bean Stew

Ingredients:

- 1 can white beans, drained and rinsed
- 4 cups chopped kale

- 1 onion, diced

- 2 garlic cloves, minced

- 4 cups vegetable broth

- 1 tsp thyme

- Salt and pepper to taste

- 2 tbsp olive oil

Instructions:

1. Heat olive oil in a pot over medium heat. Sauté onion and garlic until soft.

2. Add kale and cook until wilted.

3. Stir in white beans, vegetable broth, thyme, salt, and pepper.

4. Simmer for 20 minutes and serve.

Nutrition Information (per serving):

- Calories: 220

- Protein: 10g

- Carbohydrates: 30g

- Fat: 8g

- Fiber: 9g

- Sugar: 3g

- Portion Size: 1 bowl (about 2 cups)

Cucumber and Avocado Salad

Ingredients:

- 1 cucumber, diced
- 1 avocado, diced
- 1/4 red onion, finely chopped
- 1 tbsp lime juice
- 1 tbsp olive oil
- Salt and pepper to taste

Instructions:

1. In a bowl, combine cucumber, avocado, and red onion.
2. In a small bowl, whisk together lime juice, olive oil, salt, and pepper.
3. Pour dressing over the salad and toss gently.

Nutrition Information (per serving):

- Calories: 180
- Protein: 2g
- Carbohydrates: 15g
- Fat: 14g
- Fiber: 7g
- Sugar: 3g
- Portion Size: 1 cup

Mushroom and Barley Risotto

Ingredients:

- 1 cup pearl barley
- 2 cups mushrooms, sliced
- 1 onion, chopped
- 2 garlic cloves, minced
- 4 cups vegetable broth
- 1/4 cup white wine (optional)
- 1 tbsp olive oil
- 1/4 cup parmesan cheese, grated
- Salt and pepper to taste

Instructions:

1. Heat olive oil in a pan over medium heat. Sauté onion and garlic until soft.
2. Add mushrooms and cook until browned.
3. Stir in barley and white wine, if using. Cook for 2 minutes.
4. Gradually add vegetable broth, stirring until barley is tender.
5. Stir in parmesan cheese, salt, and pepper. Serve warm.

Nutrition Information (per serving):

- Calories: 280
- Protein: 8g
- Carbohydrates: 45g

- Fat: 8g

- Fiber: 8g

- Sugar: 3g

- Portion Size: 1.5 cups

Sweet Potato and Lentil Curry

Ingredients:

- 1 cup red lentils

- 1 large sweet potato, diced

- 1 onion, chopped

- 3 garlic cloves, minced

- 1 can coconut milk

- 2 cups vegetable broth

- 2 tbsp curry powder

- 1 tbsp olive oil

- Salt and pepper to taste

- Fresh cilantro for garnish

Instructions:

1. Heat olive oil in a pot over medium heat. Sauté onion and garlic until soft.

2. Add sweet potato, lentils, curry powder, and stir to combine.

3. Pour in coconut milk and vegetable broth, bring to a boil.

4. Reduce heat and simmer for 20-25 minutes until lentils and sweet potato are tender.

5. Season with salt and pepper, garnish with cilantro, and serve.

Nutrition Information (per serving):

- Calories: 350
- Protein: 15g
- Carbohydrates: 55g
- Fat: 10g
- Fiber: 15g
- Sugar: 8g
- Portion Size: 1 bowl (about 2 cups)

Chapter 4: Dinner Recipes

Creating a vegetarian meal plan for Type 1 Diabetes doesn't mean you have to sacrifice flavor or variety. These dinner recipes are carefully designed to be nutritious, satisfying, and supportive of your weight loss goals. Each recipe is packed with fresh vegetables, plant-based proteins, and wholesome grains, ensuring a balanced and delightful meal every night.

Eggplant Parmesan

Ingredients:

- 2 large eggplants, sliced into 1/4-inch rounds
- 2 cups marinara sauce
- 1 cup shredded mozzarella cheese
- 1/2 cup grated Parmesan cheese
- 1 cup whole wheat breadcrumbs
- 2 eggs, beaten
- 1/4 cup olive oil
- Fresh basil leaves, for garnish

Instructions:

1. Preheat oven to 375°F (190°C).

2. Dip eggplant slices in beaten eggs, then coat with breadcrumbs.

3. Heat olive oil in a pan over medium heat. Fry eggplant slices until golden brown.

4. Layer fried eggplant, marinara sauce, and cheeses in a baking dish.

5. Bake for 25-30 minutes until bubbly and golden.

6. Garnish with fresh basil before serving.

Nutrition Information:

- Calories: 320
- Protein: 12g
- Carbohydrates: 35g
- Fat: 18g
- Fiber: 8g
- Sugar: 10g
- Portion Size: 1 slice (1/8 of dish)

Chickpea and Spinach Stew

Ingredients:

- 1 can chickpeas, drained and rinsed
- 2 cups fresh spinach, chopped
- 1 onion, chopped

- 2 garlic cloves, minced
- 1 can diced tomatoes
- 1 tsp cumin
- 1 tsp paprika
- 1 tbsp olive oil
- Salt and pepper to taste

Instructions:

1. Heat olive oil in a large pot over medium heat. Sauté onion and garlic until soft.
2. Add chickpeas, tomatoes, cumin, paprika, salt, and pepper. Simmer for 15 minutes.
3. Stir in spinach and cook until wilted.
4. Serve hot with a side of whole grain bread.

Nutrition Information:

- Calories: 220
- Protein: 10g
- Carbohydrates: 34g
- Fat: 6g
- Fiber: 10g
- Sugar: 8g
- Portion Size: 1 cup

Stuffed Acorn Squash

Ingredients:

- 2 acorn squashes, halved and seeded
- 1 cup quinoa, cooked
- 1/2 cup dried cranberries
- 1/2 cup chopped walnuts
- 1 tsp cinnamon
- 2 tbsp maple syrup
- Salt and pepper to taste

Instructions:

1. Preheat oven to 400°F (200°C).
2. Place squash halves cut side down on a baking sheet. Roast for 30 minutes.
3. Mix quinoa, cranberries, walnuts, cinnamon, maple syrup, salt, and pepper.
4. Fill each squash half with the quinoa mixture.
5. Return to oven and bake for an additional 10 minutes.

Nutrition Information:

- Calories: 280
- Protein: 7g
- Carbohydrates: 50g
- Fat: 9g

- Fiber: 8g
- Sugar: 16g
- Portion Size: 1 stuffed half

Tofu Stir-Fry with Brown Rice

Ingredients:

- 1 block firm tofu, cubed
- 2 cups broccoli florets
- 1 bell pepper, sliced
- 1 carrot, sliced
- 2 tbsp soy sauce
- 1 tbsp sesame oil
- 1 tsp ginger, minced
- 2 cups cooked brown rice

Instructions:

1. Heat sesame oil in a large skillet over medium-high heat. Add tofu and cook until golden brown.
2. Add broccoli, bell pepper, carrot, and ginger. Stir-fry for 5-7 minutes.
3. Stir in soy sauce and cook for another 2 minutes.
4. Serve over cooked brown rice.

Nutrition Information:

- Calories: 350
- Protein: 15g
- Carbohydrates: 45g
- Fat: 14g
- Fiber: 6g
- Sugar: 6g
- Portion Size: 1 bowl

Spaghetti Squash with Marinara Sauce

Ingredients:

- 1 large spaghetti squash
- 2 cups marinara sauce
- 1/4 cup grated Parmesan cheese
- 2 tbsp olive oil
- Salt and pepper to taste
- Fresh basil, for garnish

Instructions:

1. Preheat oven to 375°F (190°C).
2. Cut spaghetti squash in half and remove seeds. Drizzle with olive oil, salt, and pepper.
3. Place cut side down on a baking sheet. Roast for 40 minutes.

4. Scrape the squash with a fork to create spaghetti-like strands.

5. Top with marinara sauce and Parmesan cheese. Garnish with basil.

Nutrition Information:

- Calories: 200
- Protein: 5g
- Carbohydrates: 30g
- Fat: 8g
- Fiber: 4g
- Sugar: 10g
- Portion Size: 1 cup

Vegetable Paella

Ingredients:

- 1 cup Arborio rice
- 2 cups vegetable broth
- 1 onion, chopped
- 1 bell pepper, chopped
- 1 zucchini, chopped
- 1 cup green peas
- 1 tsp turmeric
- 1 tsp smoked paprika

- 2 tbsp olive oil
- Salt and pepper to taste

Instructions:

1. Heat olive oil in a large pan over medium heat. Sauté onion, bell pepper, and zucchini until soft.
2. Add rice, turmeric, paprika, salt, and pepper. Stir to coat the rice.
3. Pour in vegetable broth and bring to a boil. Reduce heat and simmer for 20 minutes.
4. Stir in green peas and cook for another 5 minutes.

Nutrition Information:

- Calories: 280
- Protein: 6g
- Carbohydrates: 50g
- Fat: 8g
- Fiber: 6g
- Sugar: 7g
- Portion Size: 1 cup

Baked Ziti with Ricotta and Spinach

Ingredients:

- 2 cups whole wheat ziti pasta
- 1 cup ricotta cheese
- 2 cups marinara sauce
- 2 cups fresh spinach, chopped
- 1 cup shredded mozzarella cheese
- 1/4 cup grated Parmesan cheese
- 1 tbsp olive oil
- Salt and pepper to taste

Instructions:

1. Preheat oven to 375°F (190°C).
2. Cook ziti according to package instructions. Drain and set aside.
3. In a large bowl, mix ricotta, spinach, salt, and pepper.
4. In a baking dish, layer ziti, ricotta mixture, and marinara sauce.
5. Top with mozzarella and Parmesan cheese.
6. Bake for 20-25 minutes until bubbly and golden.

Nutrition Information:

- Calories: 340
- Protein: 16g

- Carbohydrates: 40g

- Fat: 14g

- Fiber: 6g

- Sugar: 8g

- Portion Size: 1 cup

Thai Peanut Tofu Bowl

Ingredients:

- 1 block firm tofu, cubed

- 1 cup brown rice, cooked

- 1 cucumber, sliced

- 1 carrot, julienned

- 1/4 cup peanut butter

- 2 tbsp soy sauce

- 1 tbsp lime juice

- 1 tbsp maple syrup

- 1 tsp ginger, minced

- 1 tbsp sesame oil

Instructions:

1. Heat sesame oil in a pan over medium heat. Cook tofu until golden brown.

2. In a small bowl, mix peanut butter, soy sauce, lime juice, maple syrup, and ginger.

3. In bowls, arrange brown rice, tofu, cucumber, and carrot.

4. Drizzle with peanut sauce before serving.

Nutrition Information:

- Calories: 380
- Protein: 18g
- Carbohydrates: 45g
- Fat: 16g
- Fiber: 7g
- Sugar: 10g
- Portion Size: 1 bowl

Veggie-Loaded Burrito Bowl

Ingredients:

- 1 cup brown rice, cooked
- 1 can black beans, drained and rinsed
- 1 bell pepper, chopped
- 1 avocado, sliced
- 1/2 cup corn kernels
- 1/4 cup salsa
- 1/4 cup shredded cheese (optional)

- 1 tbsp olive oil

- Salt and pepper to taste

Instructions:

1. Heat olive oil in a pan over medium heat. Sauté bell pepper until tender.

2. In bowls, layer brown rice, black beans, bell pepper, corn, and avocado.

3. Top with salsa and cheese, if using.

Nutrition Information:

- Calories: 360

- Protein: 12g

- Carbohydrates: 54g

- Fat: 14g

- Fiber: 11g

- Sugar: 6g

- Portion Size: 1 bowl

Lentil Shepherd's Pie

Ingredients:

- 1 cup lentils, cooked

- 2 cups mixed vegetables (carrots, peas, corn)

- 1 onion, chopped
- 2 garlic cloves, minced
- 1 cup vegetable broth
- 4 cups mashed potatoes
- 2 tbsp olive oil
- Salt and pepper to taste

Instructions:

1. Preheat oven to 375°F (190°C).
2. Heat olive oil in a pan. Sauté onion and garlic until soft.
3. Add lentils, vegetables, and vegetable broth. Simmer for 10 minutes.
4. Transfer mixture to a baking dish. Top with mashed potatoes.
5. Bake for 20-25 minutes until golden.

Nutrition Information:

- Calories: 400
- Protein: 14g
- Carbohydrates: 68g
- Fat: 10g
- Fiber: 12g
- Sugar: 8g
- Portion Size: 1 cup

Mushroom Stroganoff

Ingredients:

- 2 cups mushrooms, sliced
- 1 onion, chopped
- 2 garlic cloves, minced
- 1 cup vegetable broth
- 1/2 cup Greek yogurt
- 2 tbsp olive oil
- 1 tbsp flour
- 1 tsp paprika
- Salt and pepper to taste

Instructions:

1. Heat olive oil in a pan over medium heat. Sauté mushrooms, onion, and garlic until tender.
2. Sprinkle with flour and paprika. Stir well.
3. Add vegetable broth and simmer until thickened.
4. Remove from heat and stir in Greek yogurt.
5. Serve over cooked pasta or rice.

Nutrition Information:

- Calories: 250
- Protein: 8g
- Carbohydrates: 30g

- Fat: 10g
- Fiber: 4g
- Sugar: 6g
- Portion Size: 1 cup

Cauliflower Tacos with Cilantro Lime Sauce

Ingredients:

- 1 head cauliflower, chopped into florets
- 1 tbsp olive oil
- 1 tsp cumin
- 1 tsp chili powder
- 1 cup Greek yogurt
- 1 lime, juiced
- 1/4 cup fresh cilantro, chopped
- Corn tortillas
- Salt and pepper to taste

Instructions:

1. Preheat oven to 400°F (200°C).
2. Toss cauliflower with olive oil, cumin, chili powder, salt, and pepper.
3. Roast for 25-30 minutes until tender.

4. Mix Greek yogurt, lime juice, and cilantro to make the sauce.

5. Serve cauliflower in tortillas, topped with cilantro lime sauce.

Nutrition Information:

- Calories: 220

- Protein: 6g

- Carbohydrates: 26g

- Fat: 10g

- Fiber: 6g

- Sugar: 5g

- Portion Size: 2 tacos

Spinach and Feta Stuffed Portobellos

Ingredients:

- 4 large portobello mushrooms

- 2 cups fresh spinach, chopped

- 1/2 cup feta cheese, crumbled

- 1/4 cup breadcrumbs

- 2 garlic cloves, minced

- 2 tbsp olive oil

- Salt and pepper to taste

Instructions:

1. Preheat oven to 375°F (190°C).
2. Remove stems from mushrooms and brush with olive oil.
3. In a bowl, mix spinach, feta, breadcrumbs, garlic, salt, and pepper.
4. Stuff each mushroom with the spinach mixture.
5. Bake for 20-25 minutes until mushrooms are tender.

Nutrition Information:

*   Calories: 190
*   Protein: 8g
*   Carbohydrates: 14g
*   Fat: 12g
*   Fiber: 3g
*   Sugar: 3g
*   Portion Size: 1 stuffed mushroom

Butternut Squash and Chickpea Tagine

Ingredients:

*   1 butternut squash, peeled and cubed
*   1 can chickpeas, drained and rinsed
*   1 onion, chopped
*   2 garlic cloves, minced

- 1 cup vegetable broth

- 1/2 cup dried apricots, chopped

- 1 tsp cumin

- 1 tsp cinnamon

- 2 tbsp olive oil

- Salt and pepper to taste

Instructions:

1. Heat olive oil in a large pot over medium heat. Sauté onion and garlic until soft.

2. Add butternut squash, chickpeas, apricots, cumin, cinnamon, salt, and pepper. Stir well.

3. Pour in vegetable broth and bring to a boil. Reduce heat and simmer for 25-30 minutes until squash is tender.

4. Serve hot, garnished with fresh cilantro.

Nutrition Information:

- Calories: 320

- Protein: 8g

- Carbohydrates: 54g

- Fat: 10g

- Fiber: 10g

- Sugar: 18g

- Portion Size: 1 cup

Grilled Vegetable and Quinoa Skewers

Ingredients:

- 1 cup quinoa, cooked
- 1 zucchini, sliced
- 1 bell pepper, chopped
- 1 red onion, chopped
- 1 cup cherry tomatoes
- 2 tbsp olive oil
- 1 tbsp balsamic vinegar
- Salt and pepper to taste
- Skewers

Instructions:

1. Preheat grill to medium heat.
2. Thread zucchini, bell pepper, onion, and cherry tomatoes onto skewers.
3. Brush with olive oil, balsamic vinegar, salt, and pepper.
4. Grill for 10-12 minutes until vegetables are tender.
5. Serve skewers over cooked quinoa.

Nutrition Information:

- Calories: 280
- Protein: 7g
- Carbohydrates: 42g

- Fat: 10g
- Fiber: 6g
- Sugar: 8g
- Portion Size: 2 skewers with quinoa

Chapter 5: Snacks and Appetizers

In this chapter, you'll find a variety of snacks and appetizers that are not only delicious but also nutritious. These recipes are designed to be easy to prepare and perfect for any occasion, whether you're hosting a party or just looking for a healthy snack.

Roasted Chickpeas

Ingredients:

- 1 can chickpeas, drained and rinsed
- 1 tbsp olive oil
- 1 tsp sea salt
- 1 tsp paprika

Instructions:

1. Preheat the oven to 400°F (200°C).
2. Toss chickpeas with olive oil, sea salt, and paprika.
3. Spread on a baking sheet and roast for 20-30 minutes, stirring occasionally, until crispy.

Nutrition Information (per serving):

- Calories: 120
- Protein: 5g

- Carbohydrates: 18g

- Fat: 4g

- Fiber: 6g

- Sugar: 1g

- Portion size: 1/2 cup

Veggie Sticks with Hummus

Ingredients:

- 1 cucumber, cut into sticks

- 2 carrots, cut into sticks

- 1 bell pepper, cut into sticks

- 1 cup hummus

Instructions:

1. Arrange the veggie sticks on a plate.

2. Serve with a side of hummus for dipping.

Nutrition Information (per serving):

- Calories: 150

- Protein: 4g

- Carbohydrates: 22g

- Fat: 6g

- Fiber: 6g

- Sugar: 7g
- Portion size: 1 cup veggies with 1/4 cup hummus

Edamame with Sea Salt

Ingredients:

- 2 cups edamame in pods
- 1 tsp sea salt

Instructions:

1. Boil edamame in salted water for 5 minutes.
2. Drain and sprinkle with sea salt.

Nutrition Information (per serving):

- Calories: 100
- Protein: 8g
- Carbohydrates: 8g
- Fat: 4g
- Fiber: 4g
- Sugar: 2g
- Portion size: 1 cup

Baked Zucchini Fries

Ingredients:

- 2 zucchinis, cut into fries
- 1/2 cup breadcrumbs
- 1/4 cup grated Parmesan
- 1 egg, beaten

Instructions:

1. Preheat oven to 425°F (220°C).
2. Dip zucchini fries in egg, then coat with breadcrumbs mixed with Parmesan.
3. Place on a baking sheet and bake for 20 minutes, until golden.

Nutrition Information (per serving):

- Calories: 140
- Protein: 6g
- Carbohydrates: 16g
- Fat: 6g
- Fiber: 3g
- Sugar: 4g
- Portion size: 1 cup

Spicy Roasted Almonds

Ingredients:

- 1 cup raw almonds
- 1 tbsp olive oil
- 1 tsp cayenne pepper
- 1 tsp sea salt

Instructions:

1. Preheat oven to 350°F (175°C).
2. Toss almonds with olive oil, cayenne pepper, and sea salt.
3. Spread on a baking sheet and roast for 15 minutes, stirring once.

Nutrition Information (per serving):

- Calories: 180
- Protein: 6g
- Carbohydrates: 6g
- Fat: 16g
- Fiber: 4g
- Sugar: 1g
- Portion size: 1/4 cup

Cucumber Rolls with Avocado and Tomato

Ingredients:

- 1 cucumber, thinly sliced
- 1 avocado, sliced
- 1 tomato, sliced
- 1 tbsp lemon juice
- Salt and pepper to taste

Instructions:

1. Lay cucumber slices flat.
2. Place avocado and tomato slices on one end.
3. Roll up and secure with a toothpick. Drizzle with lemon juice and season with salt and pepper.

Nutrition Information (per serving):

- Calories: 100
- Protein: 1g
- Carbohydrates: 12g
- Fat: 7g
- Fiber: 5g
- Sugar: 3g
- Portion size: 4 rolls

Greek Yogurt Dip with Veggies

Ingredients:

- 1 cup Greek yogurt
- 1 tbsp olive oil
- 1 garlic clove, minced
- 1 tsp dill
- Assorted veggies (carrots, bell peppers, cucumbers)

Instructions:

1. Mix Greek yogurt, olive oil, garlic, and dill in a bowl.
2. Serve with assorted veggies for dipping.

Nutrition Information (per serving):

- Calories: 130
- Protein: 9g
- Carbohydrates: 10g
- Fat: 6g
- Fiber: 2g
- Sugar: 6g
- Portion size: 1/4 cup dip with 1 cup veggies

Mini Caprese Skewers

Ingredients:

- 1 cup cherry tomatoes
- 1 cup mini mozzarella balls
- Fresh basil leaves
- 1 tbsp balsamic glaze

Instructions:

1. Thread tomatoes, mozzarella, and basil onto skewers.
2. Drizzle with balsamic glaze.

Nutrition Information (per serving):

- Calories: 90
- Protein: 5g
- Carbohydrates: 4g
- Fat: 6g
- Fiber: 1g
- Sugar: 3g
- Portion size: 4 skewers

Stuffed Mini Bell Peppers

Ingredients:

- 10 mini bell peppers, halved and seeded

- 1/2 cup cream cheese

- 1/4 cup chopped herbs (parsley, chives)

- Salt and pepper to taste

Instructions:

1. Mix cream cheese, herbs, salt, and pepper.

2. Fill mini bell peppers with the cream cheese mixture.

Nutrition Information (per serving):

- Calories: 80

- Protein: 2g

- Carbohydrates: 4g

- Fat: 7g

- Fiber: 1g

- Sugar: 2g

- Portion size: 2 stuffed peppers

Guacamole with Celery Sticks

Ingredients:

- 2 avocados, mashed

- 1 lime, juiced

- 1/4 cup chopped cilantro

- Salt and pepper to taste

- Celery sticks

Instructions:

1. Mix mashed avocados, lime juice, cilantro, salt, and pepper.
2. Serve with celery sticks.

Nutrition Information (per serving):

- Calories: 160
- Protein: 2g
- Carbohydrates: 8g
- Fat: 15g
- Fiber: 7g
- Sugar: 2g
- Portion size: 1/2 cup guacamole with 1 cup celery sticks

Kale Chips

Ingredients:

- 1 bunch kale, torn into pieces
- 1 tbsp olive oil
- 1 tsp sea salt

Instructions:

1. Preheat oven to 350°F (175°C).

2. Toss kale with olive oil and sea salt.

3. Spread on a baking sheet and bake for 10-15 minutes, until crispy.

Nutrition Information (per serving):

- Calories: 50
- Protein: 2g
- Carbohydrates: 6g
- Fat: 2g
- Fiber: 2g
- Sugar: 0g
- Portion size: 1 cup

Apple Slices with Almond Butter

Ingredients:

- 1 apple, sliced
- 2 tbsp almond butter

Instructions:

1. Arrange apple slices on a plate.
2. Serve with almond butter for dipping.

Nutrition Information (per serving):

- Calories: 180
- Protein: 4g
- Carbohydrates: 24g
- Fat: 8g
- Fiber: 5g
- Sugar: 16g
- Portion size: 1 apple with 2 tbsp almond butter

Tofu Bites with Sweet Chili Sauce

Ingredients:

- 1 block firm tofu, cubed
- 2 tbsp cornstarch
- 1 tbsp olive oil
- 1/4 cup sweet chili sauce

Instructions:

1. Toss tofu cubes in cornstarch.
2. Heat olive oil in a pan and fry tofu until golden.
3. Serve with sweet chili sauce for dipping.

Nutrition Information (per serving):

- Calories: 150

- Protein: 8g

- Carbohydrates: 14g

- Fat: 8g

- Fiber: 1g

- Sugar: 8g

- Portion size: 1/2 cup

Carrot and Raisin Salad

Ingredients:

- 2 cups shredded carrots

- 1/2 cup raisins

- 1/4 cup Greek yogurt

- 1 tbsp honey

- 1 tsp lemon juice

Instructions:

1. Mix shredded carrots and raisins in a bowl.

2. Combine Greek yogurt, honey, and lemon juice, then mix
   with carrots and raisins.

Nutrition Information (per serving):

- Calories: 120

- Protein: 2g

- Carbohydrates: 27g

- Fat: 1g

- Fiber: 4g

- Sugar: 22g

- Portion size: 1 cup

Stuffed Grape Leaves

Ingredients:

- 1 jar grape leaves

- 1 cup cooked rice

- 1/4 cup chopped herbs (dill, mint)

- 1 lemon, juiced

- Salt and pepper to taste

Instructions:

1. Mix cooked rice, herbs, lemon juice, salt, and pepper.

2. Stuff grape leaves with the rice mixture and roll up.

Nutrition Information (per serving):

- Calories: 60

- Protein: 1g

- Carbohydrates: 11g

- Fat: 1g

- Fiber: 1g
- Sugar: 1g
- Portion size: 2 stuffed leaves

Chapter 6: Desserts

Desserts are the delightful conclusion to any meal, offering a perfect balance between sweetness and satisfaction. Whether you prefer fruity, chocolatey, or nutty flavors, this collection of desserts caters to a variety of tastes and dietary preferences. Enjoy these guilt-free, nutritious desserts that will satisfy your sweet tooth without compromising on health.

Baked Apples with Cinnamon

Ingredients:

- 4 large apples
- 1/4 cup chopped walnuts
- 2 tbsp raisins
- 1 tsp ground cinnamon
- 1 tbsp honey
- 1/2 cup water

Instructions:

1. Preheat oven to 350°F (175°C).
2. Core the apples and place them in a baking dish.
3. Mix walnuts, raisins, cinnamon, and honey; stuff into apples.
4. Pour water into the baking dish.

5. Bake for 30-40 minutes until apples are tender.

Nutrition Information (per serving):

- Calories: 150
- Protein: 1g
- Carbohydrates: 36g
- Fat: 2g
- Fiber: 5g
- Sugar: 28g
- Portion Size: 1 apple

Chia Seed Pudding with Coconut Milk

Ingredients:

- 1/4 cup chia seeds
- 1 cup coconut milk
- 1 tbsp maple syrup
- 1/2 tsp vanilla extract
- Fresh berries for topping

Instructions:

1. Mix chia seeds, coconut milk, maple syrup, and vanilla in a bowl.
2. Refrigerate for at least 4 hours or overnight.

3. Stir well and top with fresh berries before serving.

Nutrition Information (per serving):

- Calories: 200

- Protein: 4g

- Carbohydrates: 14g

- Fat: 15g

- Fiber: 7g

- Sugar: 6g

- Portion Size: 1/2 cup

Dark Chocolate Avocado Mousse

Ingredients:

- 2 ripe avocados

- 1/4 cup cocoa powder

- 1/4 cup maple syrup

- 1 tsp vanilla extract

- Pinch of salt

Instructions:

1. Blend all ingredients until smooth.

2. Refrigerate for 30 minutes before serving.

Nutrition Information (per serving):

- Calories: 250
- Protein: 3g
- Carbohydrates: 26g
- Fat: 18g
- Fiber: 8g
- Sugar: 18g
- Portion Size: 1/2 cup

Berry Sorbet

Ingredients:

- 2 cups mixed berries (fresh or frozen)
- 1/4 cup honey
- 1/4 cup water
- 1 tbsp lemon juice

Instructions:

1. Blend berries, honey, water, and lemon juice until smooth.
2. Pour into a container and freeze for 4 hours, stirring every hour.

Nutrition Information (per serving):

- Calories: 80

- Protein: 1g

- Carbohydrates: 21g

- Fat: 0g

- Fiber: 4g

- Sugar: 16g

- Portion Size: 1/2 cup

Almond Flour Brownies

Ingredients:

- 1 cup almond flour

- 1/2 cup cocoa powder

- 1/2 tsp baking soda

- 1/4 tsp salt

- 3 eggs

- 1/2 cup maple syrup

- 1/3 cup coconut oil, melted

- 1 tsp vanilla extract

Instructions:

1. Preheat oven to 350°F (175°C).

2. Mix dry ingredients in a bowl.

3. Add eggs, maple syrup, coconut oil, and vanilla; mix well.

4. Pour batter into a greased baking dish.

5. Bake for 20-25 minutes.

Nutrition Information (per serving):
- Calories: 190
- Protein: 5g
- Carbohydrates: 15g
- Fat: 14g
- Fiber: 3g
- Sugar: 11g
- Portion Size: 1 brownie

Coconut Macaroons

Ingredients:
- 2 cups shredded coconut
- 1/2 cup condensed milk
- 1 tsp vanilla extract

Instructions:
1. Preheat oven to 325°F (165°C).
2. Mix all ingredients in a bowl.
3. Drop spoonfuls onto a parchment-lined baking sheet.
4. Bake for 15-20 minutes.

Nutrition Information (per serving):

- Calories: 100
- Protein: 1g
- Carbohydrates: 12g
- Fat: 6g
- Fiber: 2g
- Sugar: 10g
- Portion Size: 1 macaroon

Date and Nut Energy Balls

Ingredients:

- 1 cup pitted dates
- 1/2 cup almonds
- 1/2 cup walnuts
- 1 tbsp chia seeds
- 1 tbsp cocoa powder

Instructions:

1. Blend all ingredients until finely chopped.
2. Roll mixture into small balls.
3. Refrigerate for 1 hour.

Nutrition Information (per serving):

- Calories: 120

- Protein: 2g

- Carbohydrates: 16g

- Fat: 6g

- Fiber: 3g

- Sugar: 12g

- Portion Size: 1 ball

Vegan Cheesecake with Cashew Cream

Ingredients:

- 1 cup cashews, soaked overnight

- 1/4 cup coconut oil, melted

- 1/4 cup maple syrup

- 1/4 cup lemon juice

- 1 tsp vanilla extract

- Crust: 1 cup dates, 1 cup almonds

Instructions:

1. Blend dates and almonds; press into a pan.

2. Blend soaked cashews, coconut oil, maple syrup, lemon juice, and vanilla until smooth.

3. Pour over crust and freeze for 4 hours.

Nutrition Information (per serving):

- Calories: 300
- Protein: 5g
- Carbohydrates: 24g
- Fat: 22g
- Fiber: 3g
- Sugar: 16g
- Portion Size: 1 slice

Apple Crisp with Oats

Ingredients:

- 4 cups sliced apples
- 1/2 cup rolled oats
- 1/4 cup almond flour
- 1/4 cup coconut sugar
- 1/4 cup coconut oil, melted
- 1 tsp cinnamon

Instructions:

1. Preheat oven to 350°F (175°C).
2. Place apples in a baking dish.
3. Mix oats, almond flour, coconut sugar, coconut oil, and cinnamon; sprinkle over apples.

4. Bake for 30-35 minutes.

Nutrition Information (per serving):

- Calories: 200
- Protein: 2g
- Carbohydrates: 32g
- Fat: 8g
- Fiber: 4g
- Sugar: 20g
- Portion Size: 1/2 cup

Mango Sticky Rice

Ingredients:

- 1 cup glutinous rice
- 1 1/2 cups coconut milk
- 1/4 cup sugar
- 1/2 tsp salt
- 2 ripe mangoes, sliced

Instructions:

1. Cook rice according to package instructions.
2. Heat coconut milk, sugar, and salt until sugar dissolves.
3. Mix coconut milk with rice and let sit for 10 minutes.

4. Serve rice with mango slices.

Nutrition Information (per serving):

- Calories: 250
- Protein: 3g
- Carbohydrates: 48g
- Fat: 6g
- Fiber: 2g
- Sugar: 18g
- Portion Size: 1/2 cup

Peanut Butter Banana Ice Cream

Ingredients:

- 4 ripe bananas, sliced and frozen
- 2 tbsp peanut butter

Instructions:

1. Blend frozen bananas until creamy.
2. Add peanut butter and blend until smooth.
3. Serve immediately or freeze for later.

Nutrition Information (per serving):

- Calories: 150

- Protein: 3g

- Carbohydrates: 30g

- Fat: 4g

- Fiber: 3g

- Sugar: 18g

- Portion Size: 1/2 cup

Oatmeal Raisin Cookies

Ingredients:

- 1 cup rolled oats

- 1/2 cup almond flour

- 1/2 tsp baking soda

- 1/2 tsp cinnamon

- 1/4 cup coconut oil, melted

- 1/4 cup maple syrup

- 1/2 cup raisins

Instructions:

1. Preheat oven to 350°F (175°C).

2. Mix dry ingredients in a bowl.

3. Add coconut oil and maple syrup; mix well.

4. Stir in raisins.

5. Drop spoonfuls onto a parchment-lined baking sheet and bake for 12-15 minutes.

Nutrition Information (per serving):

- Calories: 100
- Protein: 2g
- Carbohydrates: 14g
- Fat: 4g
- Fiber: 2g
- Sugar: 8g
- Portion Size: 1 cookie

Fruit Salad with Lime and Mint

Ingredients:

- 2 cups mixed fruit (e.g., berries, melon, pineapple)
- 1 tbsp lime juice
- 1 tbsp chopped fresh mint

Instructions:

1. Toss fruit with lime juice and mint.
2. Serve immediately or refrigerate until ready to serve.

Nutrition Information (per serving):

- Calories: 70

- Protein: 1g

- Carbohydrates: 18g

- Fat: 0g

- Fiber: 3g

- Sugar: 14g

- Portion Size: 1 cup

Chocolate Covered Strawberries

Ingredients:

- 1 cup dark chocolate chips

- 2 tsp coconut oil

- 1 pint strawberries

Instructions:

1. Melt chocolate and coconut oil in a microwave-safe bowl.

2. Dip strawberries into melted chocolate.

3. Place on parchment paper and refrigerate until set.

Nutrition Information (per serving):

- Calories: 120

- Protein: 1g

- Carbohydrates: 14g

- Fat: 8g

- Fiber: 3g

- Sugar: 10g

- Portion Size: 4 strawberries

Lemon Poppy Seed Muffins

Ingredients:

- 1 cup almond flour

- 1/4 cup coconut flour

- 1/4 cup poppy seeds

- 1/4 tsp baking soda

- 1/4 tsp salt

- 3 eggs

- 1/4 cup honey

- 1/4 cup coconut oil, melted

- 1/4 cup lemon juice

- 1 tsp lemon zest

Instructions:

1. Preheat oven to 350°F (175°C).

2. Mix dry ingredients in a bowl.

3. Add eggs, honey, coconut oil, lemon juice, and lemon zest; mix well.

4. Pour batter into a muffin tin.

5. Bake for 20-25 minutes.

Nutrition Information (per serving):

- Calories: 180
- Protein: 4g
- Carbohydrates: 12g
- Fat: 14g
- Fiber: 3g
- Sugar: 8g
- Portion Size: 1 muffin

Chapter 7: Smoothies

Smoothies are a fantastic way to incorporate a variety of fruits, vegetables, and other nutritious ingredients into your diet. They are quick to prepare, delicious, and can be customized to suit your taste and nutritional needs.

Green Detox Smoothie

Ingredients:

- 1 cup spinach
- 1/2 cucumber, chopped
- 1 green apple, cored and chopped
- 1/2 lemon, juiced
- 1 tbsp chia seeds
- 1 cup water

Instructions:

1. Combine all ingredients in a blender.
2. Blend until smooth.
3. Serve immediately.

Nutrition Information:

- Calories: 90

- Protein: 2g

- Carbohydrates: 20g

- Fat: 2g

- Fiber: 6g

- Sugar: 8g

- Portion Size: 1 cup

Berry Blast Smoothie

Ingredients:

- 1 cup mixed berries (strawberries, blueberries, raspberries)

- 1 banana

- 1 cup almond milk

- 1 tbsp honey

- 1 tsp flax seeds

Instructions:

1. Place all ingredients in a blender.

2. Blend until smooth.

3. Pour into a glass and enjoy.

Nutrition Information:

- Calories: 150

- Protein: 2g

- Carbohydrates: 35g

- Fat: 2g

- Fiber: 6g

- Sugar: 22g

- Portion Size: 1 cup

Mango Coconut Smoothie

Ingredients:

- 1 cup mango, chopped

- 1/2 cup coconut milk

- 1/2 cup orange juice

- 1 tbsp shredded coconut

- 1 tsp honey

Instructions:

1. Blend all ingredients until smooth.
2. Serve chilled.

Nutrition Information:

- Calories: 160

- Protein: 1g

- Carbohydrates: 32g

- Fat: 5g

- Fiber: 3g

- Sugar: 28g

- Portion Size: 1 cup

Peanut Butter Banana Smoothie

Ingredients:

- 1 banana

- 2 tbsp peanut butter

- 1 cup milk (dairy or non-dairy)

- 1 tsp honey

- 1/2 tsp cinnamon

Instructions:

1. Blend all ingredients until smooth.

2. Pour into a glass and serve.

Nutrition Information:

- Calories: 250

- Protein: 8g

- Carbohydrates: 32g

- Fat: 12g

- Fiber: 4g

- Sugar: 18g

- Portion Size: 1 cup

Tropical Green Smoothie

Ingredients:

- 1/2 cup pineapple, chopped
- 1/2 cup mango, chopped
- 1 cup spinach
- 1 cup coconut water
- 1 tsp chia seeds

Instructions:

1. Blend all ingredients until smooth.
2. Serve immediately.

Nutrition Information:

- Calories: 110
- Protein: 2g
- Carbohydrates: 26g
- Fat: 1g
- Fiber: 4g
- Sugar: 18g
- Portion Size: 1 cup

Strawberry Kiwi Smoothie

Ingredients:

- 1 cup strawberries
- 2 kiwis, peeled and chopped
- 1/2 cup Greek yogurt
- 1 tbsp honey
- 1/2 cup water

Instructions:

1. Combine all ingredients in a blender.
2. Blend until smooth.
3. Serve chilled.

Nutrition Information:

- Calories: 140
- Protein: 5g
- Carbohydrates: 28g
- Fat: 1g
- Fiber: 5g
- Sugar: 20g
- Portion Size: 1 cup

Carrot Ginger Smoothie

Ingredients:

- 1 cup carrot juice
- 1/2 cup orange juice
- 1 banana
- 1/2 tsp fresh ginger, grated
- 1 tbsp honey

Instructions:

1. Blend all ingredients until smooth.
2. Serve over ice if desired.

Nutrition Information:

- Calories: 130
- Protein: 2g
- Carbohydrates: 32g
- Fat: 0.5g
- Fiber: 3g
- Sugar: 24g
- Portion Size: 1 cup

Blueberry Almond Smoothie

Ingredients:

- 1 cup blueberries
- 1/2 banana
- 1 cup almond milk
- 1 tbsp almond butter
- 1 tsp honey

Instructions:

1. Blend all ingredients until smooth.
2. Serve immediately.

Nutrition Information:

- Calories: 180
- Protein: 4g
- Carbohydrates: 30g
- Fat: 7g
- Fiber: 5g
- Sugar: 20g
- Portion Size: 1 cup

Pineapple Spinach Smoothie

Ingredients:

- 1 cup pineapple, chopped
- 1 cup spinach
- 1/2 banana
- 1 cup water
- 1 tsp honey

Instructions:

1. Blend all ingredients until smooth.
2. Serve chilled.

Nutrition Information:

- Calories: 100
- Protein: 2g
- Carbohydrates: 25g
- Fat: 0.5g
- Fiber: 4g
- Sugar: 18g
- Portion Size: 1 cup

Chocolate Banana Protein Smoothie

Ingredients:

- 1 banana
- 1 tbsp cocoa powder
- 1 cup milk (dairy or non-dairy)
- 1 scoop protein powder
- 1 tsp honey

Instructions:

1. Blend all ingredients until smooth.
2. Serve immediately.

Nutrition Information:

- Calories: 220
- Protein: 15g
- Carbohydrates: 30g
- Fat: 5g
- Fiber: 4g
- Sugar: 20g
- Portion Size: 1 cup

Raspberry Chia Smoothie

Ingredients:

- 1 cup raspberries
- 1 banana
- 1 cup almond milk
- 1 tbsp chia seeds
- 1 tsp honey

Instructions:

1. Blend all ingredients until smooth.
2. Serve chilled.

Nutrition Information:

- Calories: 160
- Protein: 3g
- Carbohydrates: 32g
- Fat: 5g
- Fiber: 8g
- Sugar: 20g
- Portion Size: 1 cup

Avocado Mint Smoothie

Ingredients:

- 1/2 avocado
- 1/2 cup mint leaves
- 1 banana
- 1 cup almond milk
- 1 tsp honey

Instructions:

1. Blend all ingredients until smooth.
2. Serve immediately.

Nutrition Information:

- Calories: 190
- Protein: 3g
- Carbohydrates: 30g
- Fat: 8g
- Fiber: 6g
- Sugar: 18g
- Portion Size: 1 cup

Papaya Lime Smoothie

Ingredients:

- 1 cup papaya, chopped
- 1/2 lime, juiced
- 1/2 banana
- 1 cup coconut water
- 1 tsp honey

Instructions:

1. Blend all ingredients until smooth.
2. Serve chilled.

Nutrition Information:

- Calories: 120
- Protein: 2g
- Carbohydrates: 28g
- Fat: 1g
- Fiber: 4g
- Sugar: 20g
- Portion Size: 1 cup

Apple Pie Smoothie

Ingredients:

- 1 apple, cored and chopped
- 1/2 cup Greek yogurt
- 1/2 tsp cinnamon
- 1 cup almond milk
- 1 tsp honey

Instructions:

1. Blend all ingredients until smooth.
2. Serve immediately.

Nutrition Information:

- Calories: 150
- Protein: 5g
- Carbohydrates: 30g
- Fat: 2g
- Fiber: 4g
- Sugar: 22g
- Portion Size: 1 cup

Watermelon Basil Smoothie

Ingredients:

- 1 cup watermelon, chopped
- 1/4 cup fresh basil leaves
- 1/2 lime, juiced
- 1 cup water
- 1 tsp honey

Instructions:

1. Blend all ingredients until smooth.
2. Serve chilled.

Nutrition Information:

- Calories: 80
- Protein: 1g
- Carbohydrates: 20g
- Fat: 0.5g
- Fiber: 1g
- Sugar: 18g
- Portion Size: 1 cup

CONCLUSION

Congratulations on completing the "Type 1 Diabetes Vegetarian Meal Plan for Weight Loss"! Embarking on this journey has been a significant step towards better health and well-being. Over the past month, you've explored a variety of delicious and nutritious vegetarian meals specifically designed to support your unique health needs. Reflecting on your progress, it's clear that adopting a thoughtful and well-balanced diet can profoundly impact your blood sugar management, energy levels, and overall quality of life.

Maintaining Healthy Habits

The recipes and meal plans you've experienced are more than just a temporary solution; they are the foundation for long-term health. Consistency is key to maintaining the positive changes you've achieved. Keep integrating these nutritious meals into your daily routine, and continue to experiment with new recipes to keep your meals exciting and satisfying. Remember, healthy eating is a lifestyle, not a diet. Staying mindful of portion sizes, carbohydrate intake, and balanced nutrition will help you maintain your weight loss and manage your diabetes effectively.

Adapting the Meal Plan for Long-Term Success

While this book provided a structured 30-day meal plan, it's essential to adapt these guidelines to fit your lifestyle and preferences. Customize your meal plans based on seasonal produce, personal tastes, and any new dietary information you discover. Stay connected with your healthcare team to ensure your nutritional choices align with your medical needs. Embrace flexibility, and don't be afraid to make adjustments that keep you motivated and satisfied.

Final Thoughts

This book has equipped you with the knowledge and tools to make informed dietary choices that support your health goals. By embracing a vegetarian diet rich in whole foods, you've taken a proactive step towards managing your diabetes and achieving sustainable weight loss. Remember, every meal is an opportunity to nourish your body and support your well-being. Stay committed, stay inspired, and continue to prioritize your health. Your journey is just beginning, and with the right mindset and resources, you have the power to thrive.